T0280741

Cambridge Elements ≡

Elements of Improving Quality and Safety in Healthcare
edited by
Mary Dixon-Woods,* Katrina Brown,* Sonja Marjanovic,†
Tom Ling,† Ellen Perry,* and Graham Martin*
*THIS Institute (The Healthcare Improvement Studies Institute)
†RAND Europe

CO-PRODUCING AND CO-DESIGNING

Glenn Robert,[1] Louise Locock,[2] Oli Williams,[1]

Jocelyn Cornwell,[3] Sara Donetto,[1] and

Joanna Goodrich[1,3]

[1] *Florence Nightingale Faculty of Nursing, Midwifery & Palliative Care, King's College London*
[2] *Health Services Research Unit, University of Aberdeen*
[3] *The Point of Care Foundation*

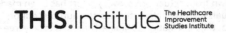
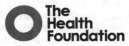

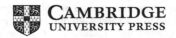

CAMBRIDGE
UNIVERSITY PRESS

University Printing House, Cambridge CB2 8BS, United Kingdom

One Liberty Plaza, 20th Floor, New York, NY 10006, USA

477 Williamstown Road, Port Melbourne, VIC 3207, Australia

314–321, 3rd Floor, Plot 3, Splendor Forum, Jasola District Centre,
New Delhi – 110025, India

103 Penang Road, #05–06/07, Visioncrest Commercial, Singapore 238467

Cambridge University Press is part of the University of Cambridge.

It furthers the University's mission by disseminating knowledge in the pursuit of
education, learning, and research at the highest international levels of excellence.

www.cambridge.org
Information on this title: www.cambridge.org/9781009237031
DOI: 10.1017/9781009237024

When citing this work, please include a reference to the DOI 10.1017/9781009237024

First published 2022

A catalogue record for this publication is available from the British Library.

ISBN 978-1-009-23703-1 Paperback
ISSN 2754-2912 (online)
ISSN 2754-2904 (print)

Cambridge University Press has no responsibility for the persistence or accuracy of
URLs for external or third-party internet websites referred to in this publication
and does not guarantee that any content on such websites is, or will remain,
accurate or appropriate.

Every effort has been made in preparing this Element to provide accurate and up-to-date
information that is in accord with accepted standards and practice at the time of publication. Although case histories are drawn from actual cases, every effort has been made to
disguise the identities of the individuals involved. Nevertheless, the authors, editors, and
publishers can make no warranties that the information contained herein is totally free from
error, not least because clinical standards are constantly changing through research and
regulation. The authors, editors, and publishers therefore disclaim all liability for direct or
consequential damages resulting from the use of material contained in this Element.
Readers are strongly advised to pay careful attention to information provided by the
manufacturer of any drugs or equipment that they plan to use.

Co-Producing and Co-Designing

Elements of Improving Quality and Safety in Healthcare

DOI: 10.1017/9781009237024
First published online: August 2022

Glenn Robert,[1] Louise Locock,[2] Oli Williams,[1] Jocelyn Cornwell,[3]
Sara Donetto,[1] and Joanna Goodrich[1,3]
[1] *Florence Nightingale Faculty of Nursing, Midwifery & Palliative Care, King's College London*
[2] *Health Services Research Unit, University of Aberdeen*
[3] *The Point of Care Foundation*
Author for correspondence: Glenn Robert, glenn.robert@kcl.ac.uk

Abstract: Many healthcare improvement approaches originated in manufacturing, where end users are framed as consumers. But in healthcare, greater recognition of the complexity of relationships between patients, staff, and services (beyond a provider–consumer exchange) is generating new insights and approaches to healthcare improvement informed directly by patient and staff experience. Co-production sees patients as active contributors to their own health and explores how interactions with staff and services can best be supported. Co-design is a related but distinct creative process where patients and staff work in partnership to improve services or develop interventions. Both approaches are promoted for their technocratic benefits (better experiences, more effective and safer services) and democratic rationales (enabling inclusivity and equity), but the evidence base remains limited. This Element explores the origins of co-production and co-design, the development of approaches in healthcare, and associated challenges; in reviewing the evidence, it highlights the implications for practice and research. This title is also available as Open Access on Cambridge Core.

Keywords: accelerated experience-based co-design, co-production, co-design, experience-based co-design, EBCD

ISBNs: 9781009237031 (PB), 9781009237024 (OC)
ISSNs: 2754-2912 (online), 2754-2904 (print)

Contents

1 Introduction

The values and assumptions intrinsic to healthcare improvement are coming under greater scrutiny.[1,2] Many healthcare improvement approaches originated in the manufacturing sector where ideas of products and customers typically dominate. However, a belated recognition has emerged that patients are not simply consumers, but instead are active contributors to their own health and to healthcare experiences and outcomes.[2] At the heart of a conscious reframing of relationships between users and providers of healthcare services lies the prefix 'co'. In this Element, we consider two major approaches: co-production and co-design. Both are commonly promoted for their technocratic benefits – such as enhancing patient (and staff) experience – as well as their potential for improving quality (e.g. clinical effectiveness and patient safety). However, as we shall show, the origins of both are rooted in broader democratic rationales.[3–5]

We begin by briefly summarising the concepts of co-production and co-design (Section 2) and how they are used in healthcare improvement (Section 3). We use examples to illustrate key issues, but do not intend them necessarily to be representative or typical. We then describe challenges and critiques relating to the implementation of the two approaches (Section 4), before outlining the current evidence base for each (Section 5). This Element concludes with suggestions for future directions in both practice and research (Section 6). Throughout, we discuss co-design in slightly more depth than co-production, as the former has a longer history of being applied as an approach to improving healthcare. However, we also highlight the potential implications of broader arguments for the latter as an important and revealing lens through which to practise and study healthcare improvement.

2 What Are Co-production and Co-design?

Though the terms 'co-production' and 'co-design' are often used interchangeably, they are not the same and have distinct origins and features. Co-production is used to recognise the two-way nature of services, that is, how the relationships and interactions between those providing and using a service influence the delivery, value, and outcomes of that service. The roles and responsibilities of service providers and users may vary, as may the degree to which the different parties consciously co-produce.[6,7] For example, shared decision-making is one form of co-production where a patient is encouraged to work with their clinician to select appropriate treatments or management options.[8] In contrast, co-design is always an intentionally applied process, used as a creative way of understanding experiences and improving services through the adoption of a range of design methods, tools, and processes that are often described as 'human-centred'. Co-design does not necessarily (or even typically) lead to users making an ongoing contribution to the delivery of services.

Although they are different, co-production and co-design have important similarities in their efforts to enable patients, families, citizens, and staff to work together in new ways, which is why we consider them alongside one another here. For instance, the principles of co-production (equality, diversity, accessibility, and reciprocity[9]) and the human-centred principles of co-design are enacted through similar mechanisms, such as dialogue, empathy, creativity, and self-efficacy.

2.1 Introduction to Co-production

The term co-production first came to prominence through the work of Elinor Ostrom in the 1970s. Seeking to explain variations in the delivery and outcomes of police services in the USA,[10,11] Ostrom's work showed differences in how actively citizens in different localities contributed to such services – for example, by reporting and taking precautions against crime. The concept of co-production has subsequently been applied to healthcare to emphasise that patients can and do play an active role not only in *producing* their own health, but also in influencing the delivery and outcomes of services.[2]

Interest in co-production has waxed and waned over the past five decades. At times, it appeared out of step with market-inspired reforms of the public sector, where citizens are cast as consumers. Today there are multiple, and sometimes contested, definitions, which has led to co-production being described as a 'fragmented set of activities, expectations and rationales'[12] used in various ways. Such ambiguities as to what constitutes co-production have led to significant variations in practice. What unites many is a recognition that users create value through their interaction with services and that organisations co-produce this with them.[7,13,14] In contrast, when applied in health services research specifically, the term is sometimes used to describe the co-production of research-informed knowledge through the engagement of policy-makers and practitioners with researchers (but, importantly, not necessarily with patients and service users).[15,16] That is not the focus here. Rather, in this Element, we think about co-production in two ways:

- as an inherent feature of healthcare. Because care is relational, service delivery is to varying degrees inevitably shaped by the interactions between patients and staff
- as a means through which to address traditional hierarchies of power and enable patients to work together with staff to improve the design and delivery of healthcare services.

In a healthcare context, Batalden et al. recognise that both of these ways of thinking about co-production are relevant: 'healthcare services are always co-produced by patients and professionals in systems that support and constrain effective partnership'.[17] Because co-production is an inherent property of any system of care, not an add-on or discretionary element, the challenge is to create 'new opportunities for innovation and improvement' around which change and improvement interventions can be planned, implemented, and evaluated.[17] Proponents of these new ways of improving quality and safety argue that direct and meaningful input by citizens and service users is needed to shape services that are of consequence to them. This, it is proposed, can lead to better value in terms of improved quality and/or quantity of services, reflecting the needs and preferences of those who support and rely upon them.[18,19]

2.2 Introduction to Co-design

Co-design can be described both as a specific category of activity within co-production[13,20,21] and as 'a conscious and voluntary act . . . concerned with how to create capacity within public service delivery systems and to improve the design and delivery of a public service'.[13] The approach originated in the participatory design movement in Scandinavia in the 1970s.[22] In a series of workplace technology projects, computer scientists and information systems design researchers took the view that 'the people destined to use the system [must] play a critical role in designing it'.[23] These projects drew on creative and practical methods to support a wide range of people to collaboratively identify and develop solutions to problems.[24] From these beginnings – and through subsequent developments in interaction, user-centred, and human-centred design (among others)[22] – design work and research[25,26] have begun to focus on healthcare.[27]

One contemporary way of explaining and visualising the design process is the Double Diamond (Figure 1),[28] which was developed by the Design Council in 2005. The Double Diamond was influenced by earlier work on creative problem-solving[29,30] (see also the Element on design creativity[31]). It remains a popular tool for explaining design to non-designers,[32] with the two diamonds representing a process of exploring an issue more widely or deeply (divergent thinking) and then taking focused action (convergent thinking). The first diamond is intended to help people understand, rather than simply assume, the nature of a problem – for example, through speaking to and spending time with those who are affected by the issues. The insights gathered may help to define the challenge in a different way. The second diamond encourages possible answers to the now more clearly defined problem, seeking inspiration from

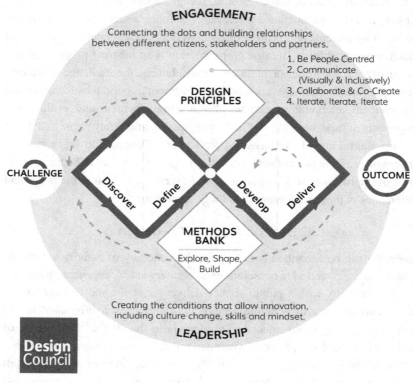

Figure 1 The Design Council's Double Diamond[28]
© Design Council 2019

elsewhere and co-designing with a range of different people. Potential solutions can then be iteratively tested at small scale, rejecting those that do not work and improving the ones that do. Underpinning the various design disciplines and practices is design thinking, which is best understood as a human-centred mindset and approach to creative problem-solving, rather than simply a set of tools.[33]

The trend for greater application of design thinking in healthcare has been reinforced by the emergence of the discipline of service design.[34,35] Described as a 'human-centred, creative, and iterative approach to service innovation',[36] service design focuses on understanding human experiences and using this understanding to design better user experiences.[34] As such, new opportunities have arisen to use co-design approaches and tools to improve healthcare services.[27] Later in this Element (Section 3.3), we also discuss a distinct form of co-design called Experience-Based Co-design (EBCD), which has been specifically developed and used as a methodology for service-level improvement in healthcare since 2005.[37-40]

3 Co-production and Co-design in Action

In this section, we describe how the concept of co-production has been applied in attempts to improve quality and safety in healthcare (Section 3.1). We then provide illustrative examples of both designer-led co-design practices (Section 3.2) and EBCD (Section 3.3) in healthcare. Key resources that explore co-production and co-design approaches in more detail are suggested in Section 7.

3.1 Using Co-production in Healthcare Improvement

Co-production has become increasingly prominent over the past decade as a new way of thinking about how to improve healthcare services.[2,11,17,41,42] To date, co-production endeavours have tended to focus on either:

- modifying individual behaviours to better support patients to manage their own health
- reshaping or creating new services and/or organisational processes.

One of the striking features of co-production is its emphasis on healthcare as a service rather than a product. This is in contrast to many traditional approaches to quality improvement derived from manufacturing models. In these models, the patient–professional relationship is imagined as akin to a customer–supplier relationship.[2] Critiques have proposed that this way of thinking risks diminishing 'the nature of the human relationships between a patient and a healthcare professional, and their contribution to health'.[2]

Coulter et al.[43] and Wagner[44] identify the importance of active collaboration with and involvement of people with long-term conditions in managing their own health and care. Building on such work, Batalden et al. explain how interactions and relationships between patients and staff are shaped not only by the formal structures and processes of the healthcare system, but also by the actions of local communities and wider social forces.[17] For example, the COVID-19 pandemic highlighted that while health and social care infrastructures often limited the potential for co-producing responses to the pandemic, this did not stop people, communities, and institutions from co-producing responses to better meet community and individual needs.[45] Consistent with others,[6] Batalden et al. propose that both patients and healthcare professionals can 'shape the system' by creating value through new and ongoing interactions within this wider context. They give two examples: an initiative to train patients and professionals to enable patients to self-manage chronic pain, diabetes, depression, and chronic obstructive pulmonary disease; and the use of shared medical appointments to support effective partnership between groups of patients and healthcare professionals.[17] These examples are typical of how co-production has more generally been interpreted and applied in efforts to improve healthcare – that is, mostly focused at the individual patient level through forms of 'engagement [that] acknowledge that patients have an important role to play in their own health care'.[46]

A well-known form of such engagement is shared decision-making. Interventions to encourage or enhance shared decision-making include those targeting individual patients (e.g. decision aids, 'patient activation' measures,[47] question prompt lists, and training for patients) or healthcare professionals (e.g. educational meetings, audit, and feedback), or both.[8] This focus on individual patients co-producing care through shared decision-making has been complemented by education programmes to build patients' knowledge, skills, and self-confidence and to promote self-management behaviours (e.g. Gilardi et al.[41]).

Initiatives have also sought to enable patients to actively engage in their own care by addressing structural issues and organisational practices. One well-known example is the establishment of a self-haemodialysis service in the Region Jönköping County in Sweden – in response to patient feedback, patients were trained and provided with facilities to perform dialysis on themselves.[48] Attempts to scale up the co-production of healthcare services include the development of learning health systems (see the Element on learning health systems[49]). A learning health system recognises that 'humans are predisposed to be cooperative and prosocial and that an appropriately designed organisation can facilitate these predispositions, thereby facilitating cooperation and co-production, at scale, to improve health, care and outcomes'.[50] A few published functioning examples now exist,[50] including the collaborative community ImproveCareNow's work with children and adolescents with Crohn's disease and ulcerative colitis[51] and an initiative to develop a learning health system for palliative care.[52]

Co-production initiatives have reported some positive results but also raise questions of equity. For example, some patients may be more able to access and engage in such programmes than others,[41] and governments may use co-production to transfer the costs and responsibilities of previously publicly provided services to patients themselves.[53] Closer consideration of the rationales for co-production may help to address such concerns. But such consideration is rare, particularly in the context of improvement practice aimed at enhancing organisational processes (albeit with some exceptions[54,55]).

3.2 Co-design: Designer-Led Improvement Initiatives in Healthcare

In the past decade, several initiatives have enabled professional designers to work in a direct, sometimes embedded, way within healthcare systems and organisations (Box 1). These projects are referred to as 'designer-led' to distinguish them from design-based approaches, which are initiated and implemented by healthcare staff, academic researchers, and/or service users who have not received formal design training.

BOX 1 EXAMPLES OF DESIGNER-LED INITIATIVES IN HEALTHCARE

- At the Mayo Clinic in the USA, the **Centre for Innovation** is underpinned by design thinking and the staff members include service designers. One project explored ways to supplement existing prenatal care and provide patients and families with more ways to interact with their care team from home. The goal was to improve the patient and provider experience by designing a new model of care. A design team created 14 experiments introducing patients to new experiences and environments, such as in-home monitoring, patient-driven appointments, online communities for patients, and appointments from a distance. The team used the insights from these experiments to create a single cohesive model of care.[56]

- **Lab4Living** is a transdisciplinary research group at Sheffield Hallam University, comprising a collaborative community of researchers in design, healthcare, and creative practice.[57,58] The group applies design skills and creative practices to identify and formulate questions, build understanding, and create solutions. An example project developed a participatory design process for a supportive neck collar with flexibility to allow functional head movement for patients with motor neurone disease. Co-design workshops brought together people living with the disease, carers, clinicians, and designers to build understanding of optimal requirements for the collar. The project used participatory methods including qualitative interviews, 2D visualisation, and 3D mock-ups. A prototyping process led to a patented medical device: the HeadUp Collar.[59]

- **The Helix Centre** – an interdisciplinary group of designers, technologists, clinicians, and researchers, based at St Mary's Hospital, Imperial College London – uses human-centred design to develop clinically evaluated digital solutions for early detection of disease, effective treatment, and holistic care. An example project involved collaborating with a working group of over 30 national organisations to redesign the way in which difficult conversations about life-sustaining treatments are conducted and recorded, with a new form and process called the Recommended Summary Plan for Emergency Care and Treatment (also known as ReSPECT). A combination of design research insights and information design expertise enabled the co-design of a new plan, process, and visual device that brings the patient to the centre of emergency care decisions. To provide accessible training and support to clinicians, a new digital tool to help healthcare professionals learn about the ReSPECT process – through interactive training scenarios and discussion tips – was also prototyped and tested.[60]

One of the most comprehensively described and evaluated designer-led projects aimed to reduce violence and aggression towards staff in accident and emergency (A&E) departments in England.[61] Prior to the project, as many as 59,000 physical assaults were recorded to have occurred annually, with violence and aggression estimated to cost the National Health Service (NHS) in England at least £69 million a year in staff absence, loss of productivity, and additional security. The project used design practices to tackle this widespread and pressing healthcare priority. The design process was based on the Double Diamond (Figure 1) and involved extensive ethnographic fieldwork; multistakeholder work to establish priorities and how designers might best contribute; design work based on models, mock-ups, and prototypes; and the delivery of solutions via a toolkit and evaluation framework.

The design team collaborated with staff at the three hospitals to develop solutions aimed at improving the experience of both patients and staff, reducing anxiety, and promoting a positive hospital culture.[61] These included comprehensive information packages for patients and others, and a programme of reflective practice designed to better support NHS frontline staff to manage and learn from incidents of violence and aggression. The solutions were then piloted in two A&E departments. An evaluation found that staff and patients experienced less non-physical aggression, particularly threatening behaviour.[62] Patients' experiences were reported to have improved through clarifying the A&E process and improving the physical environment, thereby reducing frustration and potential escalation into hostility. Complaints regarding poor information and communication with patients fell by 57% (from 49 complaints during April–September 2012 to 21 complaints during the same period in

2013). A cost–benefit analysis found that the benefits of the solutions were estimated to outweigh their costs by a ratio of 3:1. Staff also reported that the project had catalysed a cultural change through prioritising and formalising initiatives to learn from and improve staff experience, which had further positive impacts. Although the project focused on patients' experiences, patients were not directly involved as co-designers throughout this designer-led change process.

3.3 Co-design: Using Experience-Based Co-design to Improve Healthcare

EBCD was developed in the mid-2000s as interest in design-based approaches in healthcare services was growing. In contrast to designer-led initiatives such as the A&E project, EBCD typically sees healthcare staff facilitating a co-design process in partnership with patients. In this section, we describe the original aims and form of EBCD (Section 3.3.1), before outlining an important adaptation to the approach (Section 3.3.2) and illustrating the use of the approach as part of the Medical Research Council framework for developing and evaluating complex interventions (Section 3.3.3).[63]

3.3.1 EBCD of Services

EBCD was initially developed and piloted in a head and neck cancer service in an acute hospital in England.[37,38] The originators were academic researchers and designers who were seeking to draw attention to what they described as 'the burgeoning and … exciting multidisciplinary field of interactive or "user centric design" and to the whole concept of "co-designing for user experience"'.[38] The aim was to highlight the three elements of good design – performance (efficiency), engineering (safety), and aesthetics (experience) – and to consider how these should be combined in the context of high-quality healthcare services.[38]

Fundamental features of the approach include a focus on the experiences of patients and staff, and the transformative potential of participating in co-design to create broader forms of value (e.g. wider health and well-being impacts). Maintaining focus on these features is seen as more important than advocating stringent adherence to a set of steps regardless of context.[40] The originators' intention was that the mindsets and behaviours that are encouraged and prac-tised through implementing the approach (e.g. perspective sharing, dialogue, collaboration, and empathy) would become part of how participants seek to improve services in the future. For this reason, the approach is typically described and represented as a cyclical process.

Box 2 The six phases of EBCD[40]

(1) Setting up the project.
(2) Gathering staff experiences through observation and in-depth interviews.
(3) Gathering patient and carer experiences (typically through 12–15 filmed narrative-based interviews).
(4) Bringing together staff, patients, and carers to share experiences of the service and identify shared priorities for improvement, prompted by an edited film of patient narratives illustrating significant 'touch-points'* of service experience.
(5) Working on identified priorities in small co-design groups of patients and staff, using design methods (typically between four and six priorities, over three to four months).
(6) Holding a celebration and review event.

* A touchpoint is a point of contact or interaction between a patient and a service.

Implementing EBCD is resource intensive. Healthcare service staff usually lead its implementation alongside their usual roles. Projects typically take 9–12 months and comprise six broad phases[40] (Box 2) that relate to core service design practices, which involve understanding the user's perspective, making things visible, managing risk through prototyping, trying things out, and iterating ideas rapidly.[64] Guidance and advice on using the approach is available via a free online toolkit.[65]

3.3.2 Accelerated EBCD of Services

Evaluation found that although practitioners found the EBCD process to be innovative and impactful, they expressed concerns that it took too long to implement.[66] The original developers responded by making purposeful adaptations to stage 3 of the usual approach (Box 2). In the resulting accelerated EBCD (AEBCD) process, the edited films are generated by drawing upon a publicly available, extensive, and growing national archive of filmed interviews focusing on people's experiences of their health-related conditions (www.healthtalk.org) rather than by conducting and editing filmed narrative patient interviews.

This important modification was evaluated in two intensive care units (ICUs) and two lung cancer services. It proved acceptable to staff and patients.[67] Using films of national rather than local narratives did not adversely affect local staff engagement and indeed might in some cases have enhanced the process; critical comments might be perceived as less threatening when they are not directly about the people or services involved, but could still be drawn on to inform a more collaborative approach. The researchers concluded that:

> *When staff – as they did in this study – volunteer the information that this is the first time in 20 years that they have really talked to patients in this way or that it is the most rewarding thing they have ever done in their careers, the full potential of EBCD to reconnect staff with their fundamental values of care and compassion is striking. Patients, too, report a different level of appreciation for staff, a belief that they will be listened to and that change is possible, and a renewed sense of trust in local NHS services.*[67]

Compared with two earlier EBCD projects in lung and breast cancer pathways, the scale of change for the accelerated process was similar. The activities resulting from AEBCD were identified and implemented more quickly and at lower cost.[67] Improvements were predominantly small-scale changes (e.g. providing clocks to aid patient orientation in the ICU) and involved redesigning team processes (providing a new private room for receiving support after diagnosis of cancer). However, a few larger-scale processes were also redesigned, including those operating between services (changing the timing of when waste was removed to avoid ICU rest times) as well as between organisations (improving the cross-site information booklet for patients transferring to another hospital for surgery).

3.3.3 EBCD of Complex Interventions

An influential and widely used framework developed by the Medical Research Council outlines five key stages in creating a complex intervention: developing, piloting, evaluating, reporting, and implementing.[63] The Medical Research Council emphasises that 'before undertaking a substantial evaluation you should first develop the intervention to the point where it can reasonably be expected to have a worthwhile effect'. EBCD and other co-design approaches are increasingly used for the purpose of developing such interventions.[68]

Box 3 describes a study that followed the Medical Research Council framework, where EBCD was used to inform the development phase of a complex intervention to support carers of family members having outpatient chemotherapy. The resulting intervention, Take Care, comprised three components (DVD, booklet, and group consultation), and its impact, acceptability, and feasibility were tested in an exploratory randomised controlled trial.[69] Encouragingly, the study processes were acceptable to both professionals and carers, and Take Care demonstrated promise in practice.

Box 3 TAKE CARE CASE STUDY, ILLUSTRATING THE USE OF EBCD IN THE DEVELOPMENT OF COMPLEX INTERVENTIONS[69]

Developing the Intervention

- EBCD was used to develop an intervention to support carers of patients undergoing chemotherapy through:
  - non-participant observation in a chemotherapy outpatient department
  - interviews with staff and filmed narrative interviews with carers
  - three co-design events with staff and carers to agree components of a support package
  - further smaller co-design meetings to refine the intervention (considering context, content, mechanisms, outcomes, and method of delivery).
- The resulting intervention, Take Care, aimed to provide information and support to carers of people about to start a course of chemotherapy. It comprised:
  - a 19-minute supportive/educative DVD
  - an accompanying booklet
  - a one-hour protocol-guided group consultation conducted by one of two chemotherapy nurses trained in group facilitation, during which carers watched the DVD and were given the opportunity to freely express concerns and ask questions.
- The DVD and booklet included information, advice, and practical tips from carers and healthcare professionals on topics including treatment side effects, the impact of being a carer and dealing with emotions, and the importance for carers of taking time out for themselves and accessing support.

Evaluating the Intervention

- Take Care was evaluated through an exploratory randomised controlled trial.
- A total of 47 carers were recruited and randomly assigned to the intervention ($n = 24$) and control ($n = 23$) groups.
  - Recruitment to the study was unproblematic and attrition was low, suggesting that EBCD improved the acceptability of the intervention and study processes for patients and carers.
  - Compared with carers in the control group, carers receiving the intervention reported a better understanding of symptoms and side effects and were more satisfied that their information needs had been met.

- Focus groups with healthcare professionals and carers confirmed these findings.
- The researchers conclude that these findings justified assessment of the intervention's effectiveness and cost-effectiveness through a fully powered randomised controlled trial.

3.3.4 Dissemination of EBCD

Since 2011, dissemination of EBCD has been supported by a free online toolkit, which provides a wide range of resources and incorporates several case studies.[65] (Some concerns regarding 'toolboxes' are discussed later in Section 4.2.4.) The toolkit is hosted by a charity that also provides regular training for healthcare practitioners interested in the approach. Through this and other dissemination mechanisms, EBCD has become an established method for achieving and studying healthcare improvement.

The ongoing dissemination of EBCD as an improvement approach is itself a case study, both of scaling up and of developing an evidence base for applying a service design perspective. In the years following the initial pilot project, the approach was adopted in healthcare settings both in the UK and internationally.[40,66] Between 2005 and 2013, at least 59 EBCD projects were implemented in Australia, Canada, the Netherlands, New Zealand, Sweden, and the UK, and at least a further 27 projects were in the planning stage.[66] More recently, projects were undertaken with mothers or caregivers of malnourished or HIV-positive children and healthcare workers in a South African township,[70] and with formerly incarcerated prisoners in Los Angeles focusing on better integrating local health and social care services to support re-entry into the community.[71]

Green et al.'s systematic review of EBCD found increasing reports in the peer-reviewed literature from 2014 onwards.[72] The majority of the 20 studies in the review were conducted in hospital settings in the UK, mostly in mental health, cancer, and paediatrics. Eleven studies listed improvement activities undertaken as part of an EBCD process; among these, the number of improvement activities implemented (per site, service, or care pathway) ranged from 1 to 38. The impressive scale of the uptake of EBCD in the healthcare sector has been ascribed by professional designers to the framing of the approach as part of the wider healthcare improvement 'movement' (rather than as one-off designer-led projects).[73]

4 Challenges and Critiques of Co-production and EBCD

The democratic ethos and promising results of co-production and co-design are not always realised. The potential for unintended or detrimental outcomes means the need for critical thinking remains – or what Dudau et al. call 'constructive disenchantment with the magic that surrounds co-design, co-production and value co-creation in public services'.[18] Challenges to implementation are common, and loss of fidelity to underlying principles can lead to disillusionment and loss of trust and, ultimately, to poor, harmful, or inequitable service design and outcomes. In this section, some of the critiques and the challenges in applying co-production (Section 4.1) and co-design (Section 4.2) in healthcare improvement are discussed.

4.1 Co-production

Having recognised that healthcare services are by their nature co-produced, this section highlights common challenges faced when planning improvement initiatives accordingly. Foremost among these are existing power imbalances between staff and patients, the risk of inadvertently increasing inequalities, and the uncritical adoption of the language of co-production without attention to its democratic rationale.

4.1.1 The Language of Co-production

A particular challenge arises from the appropriation of the language of co-production in the context of (sometimes tokenistic) patient and public involvement in service design and research processes.[5,41,74,75] While different approaches to involving patients as partners in research have considerable overlap and often similar intentions,[76] 'co-production' is also being increasingly used to describe the production of research-informed knowledge through collaborations between policy-makers, practitioners, and researchers (in the absence of service users and public contributors).[15,16] Such ambiguities disregard significant differences in processes and aims, particularly in relation to the negotiation of power.[41,77] It is argued that without clear distinctions, the field is left with a variety of 'co-' words being used interchangeably without fidelity to core principles of any given collaborative method (a phenomenon labelled 'co-biquity'[77]). This makes meaningful comparison among studies – and therefore any theory-building – difficult.[21] The outcomes may also be potentially misleading if the terms used to describe the project suggest more inclusive, equitable, or emancipatory practice than is or was the case.[77]

4.1.2 Power Imbalances

Both co-production and co-design explicitly acknowledge and attempt to redress the significant power imbalances that can exist between staff and patients. However, seeking to work in more inclusive and collaborative ways can be difficult[78] because of existing structures, traditions, and cultures that inhibit more equitable collaboration.[77,79] In a systematic review focusing solely on the healthcare sector, Palumbo suggests that conflicting priorities and beliefs between service providers and service users, as well as their different types of expertise, are major barriers to co-production.[80] In one case study, people with cystic fibrosis in Italy were encouraged not only to self-manage their antibiotic treatment at home but also to help deliver parts of the outpatient parenteral antibiotic therapy service. However, several challenges emerged, including different or conflicting staff and patient priorities, which led to:

> ... *tensions between the interest of professional regular producers intent on ensuring stability, avoiding risks, meeting commitments to cost, efficiency and quality standards versus the potential or actual contribution of the citizen co-producer in terms of ideas, expertise, knowledge and resources.*[81]

As in this case, in the absence of enabling organisational conditions and ongoing senior management support, co-produced practices can increase both the complexity and uncertainty of the care process and have negative outcomes for staff and patients.

4.1.3 Challenges to Co-producing Healthcare and Key Success Principles

McMullin and Needham specify further challenges of personalisation, expertise, and legal liability.[78] These challenges overlap with a more comprehensive list compiled by Batalden et al.[17] Box 4 provides a summary of the known challenges.

Encompassing co-production and co-design involving service users, Greenhalgh et al. conducted a review of the impact of different models of 'co-creation' for community-based health services.[82] In the review, Greenhalgh et al. define co-creation as 'the collaborative generation of knowledge by academics working alongside stakeholders from other sectors'. Their findings point to possible ways in which collaborative participatory approaches to change in healthcare might overcome implementation challenges.[82] They identify three key success principles, outlined in Box 5, though they note that societal impact is 'by no means guaranteed'.

Box 4 Challenges to co-producing healthcare

Practical Barriers

- Engaging professionals and patients as partners is often difficult and time-consuming.
- Professionals may not have the skills or experience required to work collaboratively with patients, and co-production often requires a major shift in practice.

Power and Responsibility

- It is neither possible nor desirable to share power and responsibility equally between patients and professionals in all situations.
- The healthcare system should not abandon or ignore patients who do not have the resources or expertise to partner effectively in co-producing good health outcomes.

Diversity among Patients

- Not all patients have the desire or capacity to be active participants in co-producing their health, particularly in interventions that are ad hoc or one-off participation exercises.
- Exclusion of those most in need and/or least represented in decision-making processes within healthcare systems typically reflects the inequalities in society at large.
- Partnerships between professionals and patients are dynamic, and degrees of agency shift across time, setting, and circumstance.

Competing Forms of Expertise and Evidence

- There is a common but not necessarily well-founded perception that the value of professional expertise may be diminished by transferring decision-making and caring responsibilities to patients and families.
- Challenges may arise in establishing mutual respect between healthcare professionals and patients if or when patients acquire and apply knowledge that does not conform to evidence thresholds that are respected within medical science.
- It is difficult to calculate the long-term return on investment in evaluating this fundamentally different approach to designing and delivering healthcare services.

Contextualising Standardisation

- In initiatives to standardise healthcare professional work, it is important to consider contextual variation.

Adapted from McMullin and Needham[78] and Batalden et al.[17]

Box 5 KEY SUCCESS PRINCIPLES FOR EFFECTIVE CO-CREATION IN COMMUNITY-BASED HEALTH RESEARCH

- Take a systems perspective, recognising multiple interacting entities that are emergent, locally adaptive, and self-organising, and that outcomes cannot be fully predicted.
- View such research as a creative endeavour, with strong links to design, which:
  - requires imagination, exploration, field-testing, and reflection on emerging data to move from idea to prototype to the refined output (product, process, or service)
  - places individual experience (especially that of the patient, but also of staff) at the heart of the creative design effort.
- Recognise that the process is as important as any products or services generated. This includes:
  - how the project or programme is set up and framed, including how different partners view the process
  - the nature of relationships (which require respect and reciprocity)
  - governance and facilitation arrangements, especially how conflict is managed and the style of leadership.

Adapted from Greenhalgh et al.[82]

4.1.4 The 'Dark Side' of Co-production

Fundamental to critiques of co-production are questions concerning the goals of any given project, who is involved, and who benefits from their wider adoption. Academic critiques have consequently highlighted a potential 'dark side' of co-production.[77] Projects may, for example, be inequitable in design and appeal, potentially only involving the usual suspects (already privileged population groups) and thereby further marginalising others.[77,78] The potential for value 'co-destruction' or the co-production of 'dis/value' has also been acknowledged.[83–85] These unwanted outcomes can emerge from policy-makers using the language of co-production to abdicate their responsibilities to the public by, for example, promoting self-management over resourcing adequate service provision in a context of austerity[53] and therefore potentially reinforcing existing structural inequalities.

4.2 EBCD

Several challenges have been identified when implementing EBCD and AEBCD approaches. They include resourcing projects, facilitation, leadership support, role of professional designers, fidelity to principles and mechanisms, and the political nature of the process.

4.2.1 Resourcing Projects

A rapid evidence synthesis by Clarke et al. highlights that initiating and implementing time-intensive approaches such as EBCD and AEBCD in busy clinical environments can be challenging.[86] They emphasise that sustaining formal, practical, and financial provision for staff, patient, and carer involvement at an organisational level is key to success, but none of these is straightforward. EBCD is especially at risk of being seen as costly, particularly in view of the financial pressure that healthcare organisations work under and the absence of external research (or other) funding. Locock et al. report that the two hospitals in which they tested AEBCD subsequently decided to invest in adopting co-design more widely.[67] Their study includes a detailed cost analysis that took account of the previously hidden staff-time costs of individuals released from clinical duties over the duration of this highly participatory project. AEBCD cost an average of £28,565 per service across the four services they studied (reduced to approximately £20,000 where an edited film of patient narratives already existed). This – though about half the cost of a full EBCD project – would still be a significant investment for a local improvement project if no external funds were available. Importantly, no studies have yet compared the relative costs and benefits of service co-design with those of other improvement approaches, such as Lean (for further discussion, see the Element on Lean and associated techniques for process improvement[87]).

4.2.2 Facilitation

The success of EBCD is highly dependent on the quality of the facilitation underpinning the process.[67,86] As discussed in Section 4.2.4 on the role of professional designers, EBCD is often (although not always) conducted without professionally trained designers, in part to help build internal capacity in healthcare organisations.[67] Facilitators must, therefore, be carefully selected and supported in their role. They can be trained in design methods and tools, but they also require strong interpersonal skills and an understanding of – and willingness to embrace – the creative and emergent nature of the co-design process. Some people are more suited to or more capable of working in this way than others. Facilitators benefit from participating in wider networks to learn from experiences of peers in similar roles.

4.2.3 Leadership Support

It is important to secure support from senior colleagues and management not only at initiation but also throughout all stages of an EBCD project. The importance of leadership support was highlighted in a project to improve a learning disabilities service in England.[88] On completion, participants regarded the project as highly successful. Some three years later, the facilitator was asked for her reflections on what had been achieved:

> *Ultimately, I feel that this project was one of the best and one of the worst things I did. The process itself was great, we had fun, everyone felt respected and we got really good information. The process also took us into the planning stages in a really inclusive way and we were able to give feedback on the initial changes that we made. However, this led to a period of intense frustration as the leadership was not there to continue and make a real difference which I thought then let down all the people involved. I think some of the warning factors were the lack of clear, agreed vision for the service, new leadership with a focus on keeping their heads down, not taking risks and doing what they were being performance managed on.*

This response is consistent with other evidence suggesting that a lack of sustained engagement of senior executives – and, in this case, of effective communication with community services networks – can stifle the impact of a co-production or co-design process initiated by an operational unit.[41] Similarly, from a service design perspective, there are risks that the 'siloed nature of healthcare services' may hamper the realisation of more transformative outcomes in health and social care.[89]

4.2.4 Role of Professional Designers

Though healthcare metrics are not well suited to identifying the contribution of designers,[89] some professional designers have argued that much can be lost from a co-design process that lacks trained expertise, particularly regarding creative and ideational methods.[90–92] They question the utility of popularised management versions that often equate design thinking with creativity (which is only part of a designer's work) and a 'toolbox' (without acknowledging that design-based knowledge, skills, and training support the effective use of these 'tools').[93] For example, reflecting on an EBCD project aiming to improve outpatient services for older people, Bowen et al. propose that the limited involvement of designers in generating, developing, and communicating ideas meant that participants were insufficiently involved in the co-design of the service improvements.[92] Clarke et al. recognise that the direct involvement of professional designers typically introduces new ways of thinking and working, which successfully challenges staff and patients to think about everyday processes and activities differently.[86] However, professional designers need to be recruited and resourced, and questions about how best to embed their skills and approaches remain largely unanswered.[35] For now, the most effective role for professional designers is likely to be highly contingent upon the aims, scope, and available resources of any given project as well as its context.

4.2.5 Fidelity to Principles and Mechanisms

As with any improvement approach, adaptations to EBCD may affect fidelity by compromising its underlying principles and mechanisms.[66,72] Green et al.'s systematic review of 20 published EBCD studies reports that fidelity to the activities, as described within the online toolkit,[65] ranged from 40% to 100%, with only three satisfying 100% fidelity.[72] They highlight the importance of individual interviews over focus groups when gathering experience data from patients and staff, as well as the need to limit the time between the information gathering and co-design phases. More generally, Green et al. conclude that the following may contribute to loss of fidelity:

- (mis)perceptions of the inflexibility of the approach
- barriers to implementing co-design (lack of resources, managerial support, staff turnover, logistical issues, cohort retention, and information asymmetry)
- lack of evidence demonstrating that higher fidelity leads to better service user experiences.[72]

Deviating too far from core principles in co-design – or omitting them entirely – may be problematic for processes and outcomes. The original version of EBCD includes a substantive observational phase, allowing an additional view of how staff and patients 'go about their business in real time' as well as providing context to participants' narratives and their co-design work.[37] Observation is also cost-effective in that it can generate valuable insights relatively rapidly and with little resource. The celebratory/review event is also integral to the co-design process:[66] it offers an opportunity to recognise both the concrete achievements of a project and the practices and processes that need further work or consideration, thereby contributing to project evaluation. The event further functions as an opportunity for participating staff and patients to share and discuss achievements, learning, and ongoing challenges at the end of an often emotionally demanding collaboration. As well as closure, it provides a platform for future co-design work and continuing involvement in improvement work. Problems may arise if non-participant observation or a celebration/review event are omitted, yet this does occur.[66]

Similar limitations can occur if, instead of filmed narratives, other less rich methods are used to explore the experiences of service users. For example, Mental Health Experience Co-design is an approach based on EBCD that was developed and piloted by a service user-led organisation in Victoria, Australia, which employed computer-assisted telephone interviews rather than filmed interviews.[94] More starkly, relying solely on anonymous surveys to understand experiences of patients and staff can undermine the defining features of EBCD, rendering it unrecognisable and limiting its impact.[40]

The most commonly reported struggles are with a fundamental principle of the approach: enabling patients to fully participate as co-designers.[66,67] The co-design process is deliberately intended to reimagine and reformulate the traditional roles and relationships of staff, patients, and family members. Where successful, a carefully facilitated process not only generates collective ownership of the change process but can also prompt changes in underlying behaviours and values.[66] However, if the nature of the involvement of patients and family members regresses to consultation rather than co-design, much of the transformational potential can be lost.

4.2.6 Political Nature of the Process

Iedema et al. suggest that co-design may challenge how healthcare professionals and service users typically relate to each other and so lead to new, more equitable forms of interaction.[95] But within these new relationships, value must be placed on the design process itself as providing a space for different conversations between patients and staff, and the possibility of change. In a study of a Swedish participatory design project in primary healthcare, Sjoberg echoes and elaborates on this sentiment:

> *The design process is a political one and includes conflicts at almost every step of the way . . . if the inevitable conflicts are pushed to one side or ignored in the rush toward an immediately workable solution, that system may be dramatically less useful and continue to create problems.*[96]

Additionally, it is important to acknowledge that this challenge is not an inherent flaw of working collaboratively.[77,97] Rather, it highlights how existing structures and norms in healthcare make it difficult to work in this way and often avoid potential conflict or challenge only by failing to bring together a sufficiently diverse group of people, including people who are typically marginalised. It has been said that: 'If it feels too easy, you probably aren't doing it right.'[98]

5 The Evidence Base

As set out in Section 1, co-production and co-design approaches to healthcare improvement are promoted both for their technocratic benefits (making services more efficient, safer, and improving clinical outcomes) and broad democratic rationales (making services fairer for, and more transparent and accountable to, those they are there to serve).[3–5] Given these goals, it is perhaps unsurprising that the published literature demonstrates a strong positive bias. In this section, we review the more critical evidence for co-production and co-design and consider how the value of these approaches might be explored in the future.

5.1 Co-production

The evidence base for the theorised benefits of service co-production remains relatively weak. The originator of the concept of co-production, Elinor Ostrom, herself noted:

> *Designing institutional arrangements that help successful co-productive strategies is far more daunting than demonstrating their theoretical existence.*[99]

A number of systematic reviews have analysed co-production across the public sector. Voorberg et al.'s review of studies between 1987 and 2013 found that the studies were limited to identifying influential factors or creating general study classifications, with hardly any attention paid to outcomes, impacts, or benefits.[100] Others have drawn similar conclusions regarding the paucity of research. Loeffler and Bovaird remark that 'the actual and potential impact of co-production on citizen outcomes is as yet only sketchily researched'.[101]

Historically, studies have explored single projects and focused on motivations for participating in co-production of a public service, or they have explored barriers to co-production for both providers and users of a service. However, in the specific context of healthcare services, Gilardi et al. found little evidence – either in relation to motivations or the effectiveness of approaches –

that can shed much light on how to enhance the co-production of healthcare.[41] Most studies of co-production in healthcare settings focus on changes in the behaviour of individuals, and most use quantitative methods to assess the degree and type of patient engagement. However, a Cochrane systematic review concluded that because of the low quality of the evidence, it was uncertain whether such shared decision-making interventions are effective.[8] A small number of studies of learning health systems provide some evidence,[50,102,103] but few have explored the organisational and managerial implications of co-production.

Enhancing the evidence base presents formidable evaluation challenges. Co-production is inherently emergent, creative, and unpredictable and, consequently, it is often unclear from the outset which outcomes to measure and how. Durose et al. propose three 'good enough' methodologies that might be used to assess the potential benefits of co-production in relatively small-scale settings: appreciative inquiry, peer-to-peer learning, and data sharing.[104] Although cross-national, comparative case studies, experiments, and longitudinal studies across all sectors are underway,[21] outcomes that are perhaps less tangible but nonetheless important components of quality (including collective and long-term outcomes such as inclusivity and equity) are typically harder to link causally to co-production processes, especially within typical timelines of evaluation (i.e. conducted shortly after an intervention).

While evaluation of outcomes is important, the democratic basis and reasoning for co-production mean that even without a sound evidence base, a sound ethical rationale can be offered for co-production.[5,77] Without such an evidence base, however, arguments for the benefits that can be achieved through co-production in healthcare contexts are liable to be undermined.

5.2 Designer-Led Initiatives and EBCD

The evidence base for design-based approaches in healthcare (whether led by professional designers or EBCD) is arguably more robust than that for co-production. Here too, though, challenges remain.

Some designer-led projects have received positive evaluations, such as the earlier example of reductions in violence and aggression in A&E departments (Section 3.2). But commentators recommend that 'a programmatic approach covering a series of related studies [is required] to build legitimacy, to avoid duplication and one-off standalone studies, many of which are currently poorly reported and lack robust evaluation'.[73]

Most EBCD projects are undertaken with the aim of improving local services, are similarly small scale and heterogeneous, and typically do not undergo rigorous evaluation. However, EBCD is increasingly used in studies employing experimental methods. The first randomised controlled trial of a co-design approach (albeit one that was significantly adapted) – the Australian Mental Health Experience Co-design approach to improve psychosocial recovery outcomes (mentioned in Section 4.2.5) – found no difference between the intervention and control arms.[94] Several feasibility trials of co-designed interventions have been published, including the Take Care intervention described in Box 3.[69] Service design academics have, in turn, called for more robust considerations of the contribution and impact of design thinking to such work, including how non-designers apply design skills and approaches.[34,73]

Systematic reviews of EBCD in healthcare settings,[72] as well as broader reviews of the co-production of public services encompassing co-design approaches,[83,84] are starting to appear. Clarke et al.'s rapid evidence synthesis of outcomes associated predominantly with the use of EBCD or AEBCD in acute healthcare settings identified three categories of reported outcomes from 11 studies:[86]

- patient and staff involvement in the co-production or co-design processes
- the generation of ideas and suggestions for changes to processes, practices, and clinical environments that affect patient or carer experiences of a service, and (indirectly) the experiences of staff members
- tangible changes in services and impact on patient or carer experiences.

Co-design approaches have proven particularly helpful in engaging nursing staff in improvement work, overcoming lack of motivation and engagement by reconnecting them to their core professional values.[39] Greater engagement has enabled new, positive staff and patient interactions, which have helped to rebalance traditional power hierarchies to the benefit of all parties.[39,95] Clarke et al. acknowledge a 'real value placed by patients and staff on such changes in the personal behaviour, attitudes and culture of healthcare teams', but nonetheless report a lack of rigorous effectiveness and cost-effectiveness studies at both the service and system levels.[86] Disappointingly, little quantitative evidence exists of substantial improvements in patient or staff experience resulting from the use of EBCD. In some cases, it may be that commonly used patient satisfaction measures are simply too broad to identify the impact of specific changes (such as a new welcome pack for patients or a redesigned discharge process).

The essential 'active ingredients' in co-design and EBCD processes that might yield beneficial changes remain unclear. For example, which combinations of narrative interviews, observations, visualisation/films, facilitation, creative workshops, co-design work, and prototyping provide these benefits?

Process evaluations of EBCD and co-production initiatives in the healthcare context are just beginning to explore and suggest key mechanisms for positive impact. Dialogue, creativity, and enactment may all be important[105,106] and consistent with the service perspective underpinning such initiatives, as outlined.

Important questions relating to how to scale up any benefits of co-design across healthcare systems are beginning to be addressed. As part of a research process to identify an intervention for subsequent testing in a randomised trial, EBCD has been successfully adapted and used across a patient pathway spanning nine healthcare providers (including both primary and secondary care sectors) covering four distinct geographical areas in the UK.[107] In another example, the Collaborative Rehabilitation in Acute Stroke (CREATE) study (Box 6) adopted a mixed-methods approach that included surveys and behavioural mapping as well as interviews and observations.[108] Documenting tangible improvements in all four services, the authors report that transferring co-designed interventions developed using EBCD in two initial stroke services into two subsequent services (using AEBCD) was feasible. However, they also highlight how staff tended to focus on tasks that led to immediately demonstrable change rather than on considering the behaviours and values underpinning the rationale for those changes.

In summary, the evidence base includes many cases where the implementation of EBCD deviates from key principles and must be viewed critically. Improvements are needed both when implementing and when evaluating co-design efforts.

Box 6 CASE STUDY OF A MULTICENTRE, MIXED-METHODS EVALUATION OF EBCD IN INPATIENT STROKE UNITS[108]

Aims: To evaluate the feasibility and impact on patients, carers, and staff of using EBCD to increase supervised and independent therapeutic patient activity in stroke units. A secondary aim investigated methods for scaling up the impact of co-design approaches by exploring whether AEBCD could be used to transfer the interventions developed and implemented in the initial two units to two further units.

Setting: Two stroke units (acute and rehabilitation) in London and two in northern England.

Methods: A mixed-methods (interviews, observations, behaviour mapping, and patient self-report surveys) case comparison, before and after implementation of EBCD cycles.

Participants: A total of 76 staff, 53 stroke patients, and 26 family members (carers) were recruited to the evaluation. Several of these participants and additional staff, patients, and family members took part in various stages of the EBCD cycle. Across all sites, 43 co-design meetings were held, involving 23 stroke patients, 21 family carers, and 54 staff (all roles and including support staff such as rehabilitation and healthcare assistants).

Results: Co-designing and implementing interventions to increase therapeutic activity was feasible. Units one and two together co-designed and implemented more than 40 improvements over nine months. Filmed patient narratives from these units proved powerful triggers for action in units three and four where a similar number and range of improvements were implemented over an accelerated time period of six months. However, while observations and interviews confirmed use of new social spaces and increased activity opportunities, staff interactions remained largely task focused, with limited focus on prompting or enabling patient activity. Such findings echo a tendency in service design projects to place too great an emphasis on specific, observable changes (often to physical environments) rather than underlying behaviours and values.

6 Conclusions

The distinctive origins and features of co-production and co-design mean that they may be able to deliver on improvements in quality, safety, and efficiency at the same time as also generating broader, democratic forms of value (e.g. equity and inclusivity). Emerging evidence suggests that co-production and co-design can encourage new positive and productive relationships between staff and patients. The approaches may have merit in addressing several commonly identified challenges in improvement,[109] including, for example, staff engagement. Staff who participate alongside service users in these new ways often comment that this has 're-connected' them with the values that initially led them to a career in healthcare. Issues of power and dominance can and must be made explicit and discussed as part of decision-making processes.[4,110] Co-production and co-design offer ways to achieve this by potentially reconfiguring power relations for both staff and patients and creating the possibility for change,[110] though close adherence to the democratic and moral rationales central to the concepts of co-production and co-design is essential.

Such reflections and the potential for a more equitable way of undertaking improvement work suggest the field of improvement studies should broaden its definition of what constitutes value.[111] Where appropriate, this could include making decision-making processes more democratic, being more transparent about how and why decisions are made, increasing diversity of experiences and views, and designing systems that are better capable of responding to the needs and preferences of those who use or need them. Broadening the methods and scope of evaluation efforts to include such outcomes will help to avoid diluting the democratic and moral rationales for co-production and co-design. The potential for undertaking healthcare improvement work that benefits staff and patients alike should motivate appropriate adoption of such approaches and underpin a commitment to find better ways of understanding their additional value.

6.1 Implications for Improvement Practice

Box 7 summarises the most significant implications of co-production and co-design in healthcare improvement practices discussed by us in this Element and by other authors.[17,41,112]

BOX 7 IMPLICATIONS OF CO-PRODUCTION AND CO-DESIGN FOR IMPROVEMENT PRACTICE

- Think more critically about which quality and safety problems might benefit from being addressed through participatory approaches. Although primarily of relevance to efforts to improve patient (and staff) experience, such approaches may also potentially help address other dimensions of quality, such as clinical effectiveness and patient safety.
- Appreciate that democratic outcomes (e.g. increased equity, inclusivity, and diversity) have been overlooked in healthcare improvement, which has traditionally focused on technocratic outcomes (efficiency and cost-effectiveness) that are easier to measure.
- Ensure that democratic and moral imperatives are accounted for in improvement practices, extending beyond just the short-term priorities of healthcare organisations.
- Remember to:
  - recognise the importance of building trust with staff and patients, and be aware that this takes time
  - ensure training/education models prepare staff and patients for working in the empathetic and equitable ways that co-production and co-design encourage and rely upon, and address any staff and patient anxieties so they can collaborate in genuine partnerships

- tailor approaches to local contexts with emergent rather than fully planned strategies, whilst remaining faithful to underpinning principles
- use and help refine available training resources (see Section 7) to guide, inform, and enhance practices
- encourage facilitators to draw on relevant expertise (e.g. professional designers and community organisers)
- encourage and directly support citizens in local communities with relevant experience to contribute to improvement processes
- secure leadership support for these approaches and ways of thinking to ensure that appropriate resources are allocated, the fundamentals are not overlooked, the processes are not subordinated, or subsequent recommendations are implemented.

6.2 A Future Research Agenda

Despite growing interest in both co-production and co-design, the relevant academic literature is dominated by descriptive summaries, reports, and commentaries rather than by research studies or evaluations.[86] Box 8 presents key research priorities in co-design and co-production.

BOX 8 RESEARCH RECOMMENDATIONS

- Develop and fund longitudinal, multidisciplinary research programmes that move beyond single case studies of co-production and co-design, and include comparisons of the costs and benefits of these and other approaches to improving quality and safety.
- Investigate how the inherently co-produced nature of healthcare can inform future change or improvement interventions.
- Develop and test methodological approaches for studying and measuring broader notions of social and political value (e.g. trust, empowerment, equity); recognise that the full range of evaluation methods (i.e. methods beyond randomised controlled trials) have a vital place in assessing these ways of working.
- Evaluate the impact of staff participation in co-production and co-design (e.g. on engagement, morale, motivation, and staff well-being).

- Critically assess different approaches in co-design practices and co-production processes that seek to mobilise and equalise power relations among participants.
- Explore which 'publics' are being engaged and/or excluded by current practices, how these practices affect social inequalities, and their ethical and political implications.
- Explore how government funding, regulation, and evaluation of third sector organisations affect co-design and co-production processes.
- Form, develop, and explore collaborations and partnerships between healthcare organisations and community-led, patient-led, and user-led organisations.
- Further explore how, if at all, these approaches can be scaled up. Are they necessarily always service-specific, context-bound, and local?

7 Further Reading

Co-production

- Batalden et al.[17] – an overview of the origins and evolution of the concept of co-production, outlining how it might be applied to the work of improving healthcare services.
- A number of online networks encourage and support the co-production of public services generally and within the healthcare sector.
  - In the UK, the Co-production Network for Wales[113] and the Scottish Co-production Network[114] provide opportunities to share case studies, lessons, and resources from co-production practices and projects across the public sector.
  - Specific to healthcare, the Health Foundation hosts a co-production Special Interest Group,[115] and the International Coproduction Health Network[116] is a collaborative learning system to support existing and new communities of practice in this area of improvement studies.
- Loeffler and Bovaird[117] – an edited handbook that provides a comprehensive and authoritative account of the movement towards co-production of public services and outcomes.
- Brandsen et al.[21] – an edited collection offering a theoretical and empirical examination of the concepts of co-production and co-creation and their application in practice across the public sector.

Co-design and EBCD

- Sanders and Stappers[25,26] – explores the evolution in design research from a user-centred approach to co-designing, and provides a toolbox of generative research methods, creative tools, and techniques.
- Sangiorgi and Prendiville[35] – an edited, international collection that maps the field of service design and identifies key issues for practitioners and researchers.
- IDEO.org[118] – a design kit providing a comprehensive compendium of human-centred design tools.
- The Point of Care Foundation's EBCD toolkit[65] – a toolkit with accompanying case studies that provides a guide on how to use EBCD to improve experiences of healthcare.
- Robert et al.[40] – a brief introduction to EBCD with illustrative case studies and testimonies from patients and healthcare professionals.

Contributors

All the authors helped conceptualise the Element. Glenn Robert wrote the original draft and coordinated the preparation of the manuscript. Louise Locock, Oli Williams, Jocelyn Cornwell, Sara Donetto, and Joanna Goodrich contributed to the review and revisions of the original draft, providing critical commentaries and edits. All authors have approved the final version.

Conflicts of Interest

Through the Point of Care Foundation, Jocelyn Cornwell and Joanna Goodrich provide training in the EBCD approach for practitioners and seminars for doctoral and postdoctoral students; Glenn Robert has previously contributed to the training and seminars. Jocelyn Cornwell is a member of the engagement and involvement advisory board for THIS Institute (The Healthcare Improvement Studies Institute). Louise Locock, Oli Williams, and Sara Donetto have no conflicts of interest.

Acknowledgements

We thank the peer reviewers for their insightful comments and recommendations to improve this Element. A list of peer reviewers is published at www.cambridge.org/IQ-peer-reviewers.

Funding

This Element was funded by THIS Institute (www.thisinstitute.cam.ac.uk). THIS Institute is strengthening the evidence base for improving the quality and safety of healthcare. THIS Institute is supported by a grant to the University of Cambridge from the Health Foundation – an independent charity committed to bringing about better health and healthcare for people in the UK. Glenn Robert, Oli Williams, and Sara Donetto are affiliated to the Samskapa research programme on co-production led by Jönköping University. This is funded by Forte, the Swedish Research Council for Health, Working Life and Welfare under grant agreement no. 2018–01431. Oli Williams is supported by the Health Foundation's grant to the University of Cambridge for THIS Institute.

About the Authors

Glenn Robert is Professor at King's College London. His research draws on the fields of organisational studies and organisational sociology, and incorporates the study of innovations in the organisation and delivery of healthcare services as well as quality improvement interventions.

Louise Locock is Professor in Health Services Research at the University of Aberdeen. Her research interests include personal experience of health and illness, patient-centred quality improvement and co-design, and patient and family involvement in research and care, and focusing recently on better use of patient experience data to improve care.

Oli Williams is a THIS Institute postdoctoral fellow at King's College London, and he previously received the NIHR CLAHRC West Dan Hill Fellowship in Health Equity. He is a sociologist and his research focuses on health inequalities, the promotion of healthy lifestyles, obesity, weight stigma, equitable intervention, and co-production.

Jocelyn Cornwell is the former Chief Executive of The Point of Care Foundation. She worked in health regulation, first at the Audit Commission and then at the Commission for Health Improvement. She now chairs the board of trustees of Action against Medical Accidents (AvMA).

Sara Donetto is a social scientist with a background in medicine and a senior lecturer at King's College London. Her research interests include pedagogical innovation in healthcare professional education, critical understandings of person-centred and relationship-centred care, and patient and staff experiences of care.

Joanna Goodrich is Research Associate at the Cicely Saunders Institute. She joined King's College London in 2020, having worked for many years in the not-for-profit sector on health service policy and improvement, most recently at The Point of Care Foundation. Her research interests include patient experience, EBCD, healthcare staff experience, and quality improvement.

Creative Commons Licence

References

1. Dixon-Woods M. How to improve healthcare improvement – an essay by Mary Dixon-Woods. *BMJ* 2019; 366: l5514. https://doi.org/10.1136/bmj.l5514.

2. Batalden P. Getting more health from healthcare: quality improvement must acknowledge patient coproduction – an essay by Paul Batalden. *BMJ* 2018; 1: k3617. https://doi.org/10.1136/bmj.k3617.

3. Verschuere B, Vanleene D, Steen T, Brandsen T. Democratic co-production: concepts and determinants. In: Brandsen T, Steen T, Verschuere B, editors. *Co-Production and Co-Creation: Engaging Citizens in Public Services*. New York: Routledge; 2018: 243–51. https://doi.org/10.4324/9781315204956.

4. Farr M. Power dynamics and collaborative mechanisms in co-production and co-design processes. *Crit Soc Policy* 2018; 38: 623–44. https://doi.org/10.1177/0261018317747444.

5. Williams O, Robert G, Martin GP, Hanna E, O'Hara J. Is co-production just really good PPI? Making sense of patient and public involvement and co-production networks. In: Bevir M, Waring J, editors. *Decentring Health and Care Networks*. London: Palgrave; 2020: 213–37. https://doi.org/10.1007/978-3-030-40889-3.

6. Osborne SP, Radnor Z, Strokosch K. Co-production and the co-creation of value in public services: a suitable case for treatment? *Public Manage Rev* 2016; 18: 639–53. https://doi.org/10.1080/14719037.2015.1111927.

7. Fugini M, Bracci E, Sicilia M, editors. *Co-production in the Public Sector. Experiences and Challenges*. Springer; 2016. https://doi.org/10.1007/978-3-319-30558-5.

8. Légaré F, Adekpedjou R, Stacey D, et al. Interventions for increasing the use of shared decision making by healthcare professionals. *Cochrane Database Syst Rev* 2018; 7: CD006732. https://doi.org/10.1002/14651858.CD006732.pub4.

9. Social Care Institute for Excellence. Co-production in social care: what it is and how to do it. www.scie.org.uk/publications/guides/guide51/what-is-coproduction/principles-of-coproduction.asp (accessed 17 February 2022).

10. Ostrom E, Parks RB, Whitaker GP, et al. The public service production process: a framework for analyzing police services. *Policy Stud J* 1978; 7: 381–9. https://doi.org/10.1111/j.1541-0072.1978.tb01782.x.

11. Brudney JL, England RE. Toward a definition of the coproduction concept. *Publ Admin Rev* 1983; 43: 59–65. https://doi.org/:10.2307/975300.

12. Ewert B, Evers A. An ambiguous concept: on the meanings of co-production for health care users and user organizations. *VOLUNTAS: Int J Volunt Nonprofit Organizations* 2014; 25: 425–42. https://doi.org/10.1007/s11266-012-9345-2.
13. Osborne SP, Radnor Z, Nasi G. A new theory for public service management? Toward a (public) service-dominant approach. *Am Rev Pub Adm* 2012; 43: 135–58. https://doi.org/10.1177/0275074012466935.
14. Osborne SP, Strokosch K. It takes two to tango? Understanding the co-production of public services by integrating the services management and public administration perspectives. *Brit J Manage* 2013; 24: S31–S47. https://doi.org/10.1111/1467-8551.12010.
15. Marshall M, Davies H, Ward V, et al. Optimising the impact of health services research on the organisation and delivery of health services: a mixed-methods study. *Health Soc Care Deliv Res* 2022; 10(3). https://doi.org/10.3310/HFUU3193.
16. Martin S. Co-production of social research: strategies for engaged scholarship. *Publ Money Manag* 2010; 30: 211–18. https://doi.org/10.1080/09540962.2010.492180.
17. Batalden M, Batalden P, Margolis P, et al. Coproduction of healthcare service. *BMJ Qual Saf* 2016; 25: 509–17. http://dx.doi.org/10.1136/bmjqs-2015-004315.
18. Dudau A, Glennon R, Verschuere B. Following the yellow brick road? (Dis)enchantment with co-design, co-production and value co-creation in public services. *Public Manage Rev* 2019; 21: 1577–94. https://doi.org/10.1080/14719037.2019.1653604.
19. Parks RB, Baker PC, Kiser L, et al. Consumers as coproducers of public services: some economic and institutional considerations. *Policy Stud J* 1981; 9: 1001–11. https://doi.org/10.1111/j.1541-0072.1981.tb01208.x.
20. Bovaird T, Loeffler E. We're all in this together: harnessing user and community co-production of public outcomes. In: Staite C, editor. *Making Sense of the Future: Do We Need a New Model of Public Services?* Birmingham: Institute of Local Government Studies, University of Birmingham; 2013. www.birmingham.ac.uk/Documents/college-social-sciences/government-society/inlogov/publications/2013/chapter-4-bovaird-loeffler.pdf (accessed 17 February 2022).
21. Brandsen T, Steen T, Verschuere B, editors. *Co-Production and Co-Creation: Engaging Citizens in Public Services.* New York: Routledge; 2018. https://doi.org/10.4324/9781315204956.
22. Robert G, Donetto S, Williams O. Co-designing healthcare services with patients. In: Loeffler E, Bovaird T, editors. *The Palgrave Handbook of*

Co-Production of Public Services and Outcomes. London: Palgrave Macmillan; 2021: 313–34. https://doi.org/10.1007/978-3-030-53705-0.

23. Schuler D, Namioka A, editors. *Participatory Design: Principles and Practices*. Boca Raton, FL: CRC Press; 1993.

24. Reason P, Bradbury H, editors. *The SAGE Handbook of Action Research. Participative Inquiry and Practice, 1st edition*. London: Sage; 2001.

25. Sanders EB-N, Stappers P. Co-creation and the new landscapes of design. *CoDesign* 2008; 4: 5–18. https://doi.org/10.1080/15710880 701875068.

26. Sanders EB-N, Stappers P. *Convivial Toolbox*. Amsterdam: BIS; 2012.

27. Tsekleves E, Cooper R, editors. *Design for Health*. London: Routledge; 2017.

28. Design Council. Framework for innovation: Design Council's evolved Double Diamond; 17 May 2019. www.designcouncil.org.uk/our-work/skills-learning /tools-frameworks/framework-for-innovation-design-councils-evolved-double -diamond (accessed 27 June 2022).

29. Arnold JE, Clancey WJ. *Creative Engineering: Promoting Innovation by Thinking Differently*. Stanford: Stanford Digital Repository; 1969. http:// purl.stanford.edu/jb100vs5745 (accessed 17 February 2022).

30. Archer LB. *Systematic Method for Designers*. London: Council of Industrial Design; 1965.

31. Jun T, Hignett S, Clarkson PJ. Design creativity. In: Dixon-Woods M, Brown K, Marjanovic S, et al., editors. *Elements of Improving Quality and Safety in Healthcare*. Cambridge: Cambridge University Press; forthcoming.

32. Drew C. The Double Diamond, 15 years on. Design Council; 2 September 2019. https://medium.com/design-council/the-double-diamond-15-years-on-8c7bc594610e (accessed 17 February 2022).

33. Cross N. Designerly ways of knowing. *Design Studies* 1982; 3: 221–7. https://doi.org/10.1016/0142-694X(82)90040-0.

34. Pfannstiel MA, Rasche C, editors. *Service Design and Service Thinking in Healthcare and Hospital Management. Theory, Concepts, Practice*. Switzerland: Springer; 2019.

35. Sangiorgi D, Prendiville A, editors. *Designing for Service. Key Issues and New Directions*. London: Bloomsbury; 2017.

36. Meroni A, Sangiorgi D. *Design for Services*. Farnham: Gower; 2011.

37. Bate SP, Robert G. Experience-based design: from redesigning the system around the patient to co-designing services with the patient. *Qual Saf Health Care* 2006; 15: 307–10. http://dx.doi.org/10.1136/qshc.2005.016527.

38. Bate SP, Robert G. *Bringing User Experience to Healthcare Improvement: The Concepts, Methods and Practices of Experience-Based Design.* Oxford: Radcliffe; 2007.

39. Robert G. Participatory action research: using experience-based co-design to improve the quality of health care services. In: Ziebland S, Coulter A, Calabrase JD, Locock L, editors. *Understanding and Using Health Experiences: Improving Patient Care.* Oxford: Oxford University Press; 2013. https://doi.org/10.1093/acprof:oso/9780199665372.003.0014.

40. Robert G, Cornwell J, Locock L, et al. Patients and staff as co-designers of health care services. *BMJ* 2015; 350: g7714. https://doi.org/10.1136/bmj.g7714.

41. Gilardi S, Guglielmetti C, Marsilio M, Sorrentino M. Co-production in healthcare: moving patient engagement towards a managerial approach. In: Fugini M, Bracci E, Sicilia M, editors. *Co-production in the Public Sector: Experiences and Challenges.* Springer; 2016: 77–95. https://doi.org/10.1007/978-3-319-30558-5.

42. Elwyn G, Nelson E, Hager A, et al. Coproduction: when users define quality. *BMJ Qual Saf* 2020; 29: 711–16. https://doi.org/10.1136/bmjqs-2019-009830.

43. Coulter A, Roberts S, Dixon A. *Delivering Better Services for People with Long-Term Conditions: building the House of Care.* London: The King's Fund; 2013. www.kingsfund.org.uk/publications/delivering-better-services-people-long-term-conditions (accessed 17 February 2022).

44. Wagner EH. Chronic disease management: what will it take to improve care for chronic illness? *Eff Clin Pract* 1998; 1: 2–4.

45. Williams O, Tembo D, Ocloo J, et al. *COVID-19 and Co-production in Health and Social Care Research, Policy and Practice: Co-production Methods and Working Together at a Distance* (vol 2). Bristol: Policy Press; 2021. https://doi.org/10.47674/9781447361794.

46. Coulter A. Patient engagement. What works? *J Ambulatory Care Manage* 2012; 35: 80–9. https://doi.org/10.1097/JAC.0b013e318249e0fd.

47. Hibbard J, Stockard J, Mahoney ER, Tusler M. Development of the patient activation measure (PAM): conceptualizing and measuring activation in patients and consumers. *Health Serv Res* 2004; 39: 1005–26. https://doi.org/10.1111/j.1475-6773.2004.00269.x.

48. Shinkman R. Is 'empowered dialysis' the key to better outcomes? *NEJM Catalyst*; 15 March 2018. https://catalyst.nejm.org/doi/full/10.1056/CAT.18.0232 (accessed 17 February 2022).

49. Foley T, Horwitz L. Learning health systems. In: Dixon-Woods M, Brown K, Marjanovic S, et al., editors. *Elements of Improving Quality*

and Safety in Healthcare. Cambridge: Cambridge University Press; forthcoming.

50. Britto MT, Fuller SC, Kaplan HC, et al. Using a network organisational architecture to support the development of learning healthcare systems. *BMJ Qual Saf* 2018; 27: 937–46. http://dx.doi.org/10.1136/bmjqs-2017-007219.

51. ImproveCareNow. Purpose and success; 2020. www.improvecarenow.org/purpose-success (accessed 17 February 2022).

52. Kamal AH, Kirkland KB, Meier DE, et al. A person-centered, registry-based learning health system for palliative care: a path to coproducing better outcomes, experience, value, and science. *J Palliat Med* 2018; 21: S-61–S-67. http://doi.org/10.1089/jpm.2017.0354.

53. Fotaki M. Co-production under the financial crisis and austerity: a means of democratizing public services or a race to the bottom? *J Manage Inquiry* 2015; 24: 433–8. https://doi.org/10.1177/1056492615579790.

54. Levy P. Self-dialysis in Sweden; 11 August 2011. http://runningahospital.blogspot.com/2011/08/self-dialysis-in-sweden.html (accessed 9 March 2022).

55. Tholstrup J. Empowering patients to need less care and do better in Highland Hospital, South Sweden. In: Loeffler E, Power G, Bovaird T, Hine-Hughes F, editors. *Co-Production of Health and Wellbeing in Scotland.* Edinburgh: Governance International; 2013: 90–9. www.govint.org/fileadmin/user_upload/publications/Co-Production_of_Health_and_Wellbeing_in_Scotland.pdf (accessed 17 February 2022).

56. Mayo Clinic. OB Nest: a new vision for prenatal care; 19 March 2021. www.mayoclinic.org/medical-professionals/obstetrics-gynecology/news/ob-nest-a-new-vision-for-prenatal-care/mac-20509442 (accessed 11 February 2022).

57. Chamberlain P, Mawson S, Wolstenholme D. Services: service design in chronic health. In: Tsekleves E, Cooper R, editors. *Design for Health.* London: Routledge; 2017: 216–40.

58. Lab4Living. https://lab4living.org.uk (accessed 17 February 2022).

59. Lab4Living. Head-Up: developing a novel cervical orthosis for neck weakness. https://lab4living.org.uk/projects/head-up (accessed 17 February 2022).

60. Helix Centre. ReSPECT: personalised care, even in an emergency. https://helixcentre.com/project-respect (accessed 17 February 2022).

61. Design Council. *Reducing Violence and Aggression in A&E Through a Better Experience.* London: Design Council; 2011. www.designcouncil.org.uk/sites/default/files/asset/document/ReducingViolenceAndAggressionInAandE.pdf (accessed 17 February 2022).

62. Frontier Economics. *Reducing Violence and Aggression in A&E: Through a Better Experience. An Impact Evaluation for the Design Council.* London: Frontier Economics; 2013. www.designcouncil.org.uk/sites/default/files/ asset/document/AE_FE_evaluation_report.pdf (accessed 17 February 2022).

63. Medical Research Council. *Developing and Evaluating Complex Interventions.* London: Medical Research Council; 2006. https://webarc hive.nationalarchives.gov.uk/ukgwa/20220207162925/http://mrc.ukri.org/ documents/pdf/complex-interventions-guidance (accessed 27 June 2022).

64. Burns C, Cottam H, Vanstone C, et al. *RED Paper 02: Transformation Design.* London: Design Council; 2006. www.designcouncil.org.uk/resources/report/ red-paper-02-transformation-design (accessed 17 February 2022).

65. The Point of Care Foundation. EBCD: experience-based co-design toolkit. www.pointofcarefoundation.org.uk/resource/experience-based-co-design- ebcd-toolkit (accessed 17 February 2022).

66. Donetto S, Pierri P, Tsianakas V, et al. Experience-based co-design and health-care improvement: realising participatory design in the public sector. *Design J* 2015; 18: 227–48. https://doi.org/10.2752/175630615X14212498964312.

67. Locock L, Robert G, Boaz A, et al. Testing accelerated experience-based co-design: a qualitative study of using a national archive of patient experi-ence narrative interviews to promote rapid patient-centred service improvement. *Health Serv Deliv Res* 2014; 2(4). https://doi.org/10.3310 /hsdr02040.

68. O'Cathain A, Croot L, Duncan E, et al. Guidance on how to develop complex interventions to improve health and healthcare. *BMJ Open* 2019; 9: e029954. https://doi.org/10.1136/bmjopen-2019-029954.

69. Tsianakas V, Robert G, Richardson A, et al. Enhancing the experience of carers in the chemotherapy outpatient setting: an exploratory randomised controlled trial to test the impact, acceptability and feasibility of a complex intervention co-designed by carers and staff. *Support Care Cancer* 2015; 23: 3069–80. https://doi.org/10.1007/s00520-015-2677-x.

70. Van Deventer C, Robert G, Wright A. Improving childhood nutrition and wellness in South Africa: involving mothers/caregivers of malnourished or HIV positive children and health care workers as co-designers to enhance a local quality improvement intervention. *BMC Health Serv Res* 2016; 16: 358. https://doi.org/10.1186/s12913-016-1574-4.

71. Mendel P, Davis LM, Turner S, et al. *Co-Design of Services for Health and Reentry (CO-SHARE): An Experience-Based Co-Design (EBCD) Pilot Study with Individuals Returning to Community from Jail and Service Providers in Los Angeles County.* Santa Monica, CA: RAND Corporation; 2019. www .rand.org/pubs/research_reports/RR2844.html (accessed 17 February 2022).

72. Green T, Bonner A, Teleni L, et al. Use and reporting of experience-based codesign studies in the healthcare setting: a systematic review. *BMJ Qual Saf* 2020; 29: 64–76. https://doi:10.1136/bmjqs-2019-009570.

73. Macdonald A. Products: negotiating design within sceptical territory: lessons from healthcare. In: Tsekleves E, Cooper R, editors. *Design for Health*. London: Routledge; 2017: 311–27.

74. Oliver SR, Rees RW, Clarke-Jones L, et al. A multidimensional conceptual framework for analysing public involvement in health services research. *Health Expect* 2008; 11: 72–84. https://doi.org/10.1111/j.1369-7625 .2007.00476.x.

75. Madden M, Speed E. Beware zombies and unicorns: toward critical patient and public involvement in health research in a neoliberal context. *Front Sociol* 2017; 2. https://doi.org/10.3389/fsoc.2017.00007.

76. Locock L, Boaz A. Drawing straight lines along blurred boundaries: qualitative research, patient and public involvement in medical research, co-production and co-design. *Evid Policy: J Res Debate Pract* 2019; 15: 409–21. https://doi.org/10.1332/174426419X15552999451313.

77. Williams O, Sarre S, Papoulias C, et al. Lost in the shadows: reflections on the dark side of co-production. *Health Res Policy Syst* 2020; 18. https://doi .org/10.1186/s12961-020-00558-0.

78. McMullin C, Needham C. Co-production in healthcare. In: Brandsen T, Steen T, Verschuere B, editors. *Co-Production and Co-Creation: Engaging Citizens in Public Services*. New York: Routledge; 2018: 151–60. https:// doi.org/10.4324/9781315204956.

79. Ocloo J, Garfield S, Dean Franklin B, Dawson S. Exploring the theory, barriers and enablers for patient and public involvement across health, social care and patient safety: a systematic review of reviews. *Health Res Policy Syst* 2021; 19: 8. https://doi.org/10.1186/s12961-020-00644-3.

80. Palumbo, R. Contextualizing co-production of health care: a systematic literature review. *Int J Public Sect Manage* 2016; 29: 72–90. https://doi.org /10.1108/IJPSM-07-2015-0125.

81. Schlappa H, Imani Y. Who is in the lead? New perspectives on leading service co-production. In: Brandsen T, Steen T, Verschuere B, editors. *Co-Production and Co-Creation: Engaging Citizens in Public Services*. New York: Routledge; 2018: 99–108.

82. Greenhalgh T, Jackson C, Shaw S, Janamian T. Achieving research impact through co-creation in community-based health services. *Milbank Q* 2016; 94: 392–429. https://doi.org/10.1111/1468-0009.12197.

83. Steen T, Brandsen T, Verschuere B. The dark side of co-creation and co-production: seven evils. In: Brandsen T, Steen T, Verschuere B, editors.

Co-Production and Co-Creation: Engaging Citizens in Public Services. New York: Routledge; 2018: 284–93. https://doi.org/10.4324/97813 15204956.

84. Williams BN, Kang SC, Johnson J. (Co)-contamination as the dark side of co-production: public value failures in co-production processes. *Public Manage Rev* 2016; 18: 692–717. https://doi.org/10.1080/14719037.2015.1111660.

85. Cluley V, Parker S, Radnor Z. New development: expanding public service value to include dis/value. *Publ Money Manag* 2021; 41: 656–9. https://doi .org/10.1080/09540962.2020.1737392.

86. Clarke D, Jones F, Harris R, Robert G. What outcomes are associated with developing and implementing coproduced interventions in acute healthcare settings? A rapid evidence synthesis. *BMJ Open* 2017; 7: e014650. https:// bmjopen.bmj.com/content/7/7/e014650.

87. Radnor Z, Williams S. Lean and associated techniques for process improvement. In: Dixon-Woods M, Brown K, Marjanovic S, et al., editors. *Elements of Improving Quality and Safety in Healthcare.* Cambridge: Cambridge University Press; forthcoming.

88. The Point of Care Foundation. Involving people with learning disabilities – Leicestershire Partnership NHS Trust. www.pointofcarefoundation.org.uk /resource/involving-people-learning-disabilities-leicestershire-partnership -nhs-trust (accessed 17 February 2022).

89. Prendiville A. Service design methods: knowledge co-production in health and social care. In: Pfannstiel MA, Rasche C, editors. *Service Design and Service Thinking in Healthcare and Hospital Management. Theory, Concepts, Practice.* Switzerland: Springer; 2019: 359–75. https://doi.org /10.1007/978-3-030-00749-2.

90. Langley J, Wolstenholme D, Cooke J. 'Collective making' as knowledge mobilisation: the contribution of participatory design in the co-creation of knowledge in healthcare. *BMC Health Serv Res* 2018; 18: 585. https://doi .org/10.1186/s12913-018-3397-y.

91. Thomson A, Rivas C, Giovanni G. Multiple Sclerosis outpatient future groups: improving the quality of participant interaction and ideation tools within service improvement activities. *BMC Health Serv Res* 2015; 15: 105. https://doi.org/10.1186/s12913-015-0773-8.

92. Bowen S, McSeveny K, Lockley E, et al. How was it for you? Experiences of participatory design in the UK health service. *CoDesign* 2013; 9: 230–46. https://doi.org/10.1080/15710882.2013.846384.

93. Johansson-Sköldberg U, Woodilla J, Çetinkaya M. Design thinking: past, present and possible futures. *Creat Innov Manage* 2013; 22: 121–45. https://doi.org/10.1111/caim.12023.

94. Palmer, VJ, Chondros, P, Furler, J, et al. The CORE study – an adapted mental health experience codesign intervention to improve psychosocial recovery for people with severe mental illness: a stepped wedge cluster randomized-controlled trial. *Health Expect* 2021; 24: 1948–61. https://doi.org/10.1111/hex.13334.

95. Iedema R, Merrick E, Piper D, et al. Co-design as discursive practice in emergency health services: the architecture of deliberation. *J Appl Behav Sci* 2010; 46:73–91. https://doi.org/10.1177/0021886309357544.

96. Sjoberg C. Voices in design: argumentation in participatory development. Licentiate Thesis (Thesis no. 436), Linkoping Studies in Science and Technology, Department of Computer and Information Science, Linkoping University, Linkoping, Sweden, 1996.

97. Donetto S, Cribb A. Researching involvement in health care practices: interrupting or reproducing medicalization? *J Eval Clin Pract* 2011; 17: 907–91. https://doi.org/10.1111/j.1365-2753.2011.01725.x.

98. Facer K, Enright B. *Creating Living Knowledge: the Connected Communities Programme, Community-University Partnerships and the Participatory Turn in the Production Of Knowledge.* Bristol: Arts and Humanities Research Council; 2016.

99. Ostrom E. Crossing the great divide: coproduction, synergy, and development. *World Devel* 1996; 24: 1073–87. https://doi.org/10.1016/0305-750X(96)00023-X.

100. Voorberg WH, Bekkers VJJM, Tummers LG. A systematic review of co-creation and co-production: embarking on the social innovation journey. *Public Manage Rev* 2015; 17: 1333–57. https://doi.org/10.1080/14719037.2014.930505.

101. Loeffler E, Bovaird T. User and community co-production of public services: what does the evidence tell us? *Int J Public Admin* 2016; 48: 1–14. https://doi.org/10.1080/01900692.2016.1250559.

102. Seid M, Hartley DM, Dellal G, Myers S, Margolis PA. Organizing for collaboration: an actororiented architecture in ImproveCareNow. *Learn Health Sys* 2020; 4: e10205. https://doi.org/10.1002/lrh2.10205.

103. Gremyr A, Malm U, Lundin L, Andersson A-C. A learning health system for people with severe mental illness: a promise for continuous learning, patient coproduction and more effective care. *Digital Psyc* 2019; 2: 83. https://doi.org/10.1080/2575517X.2019.1622397.

104. Durose C, Needham C, Mangan C, Ress J. Generating 'good enough' evidence for co-production. *Evid Policy: J Res Debate Pract* 2017; 13: 135–51. https://doi.org/10.1332/174426415X14440619792955.

105. Palmer VJ, Weavell W, Callander R, et al. The participatory zeitgeist: an explanatory theoretical model of change in an era of coproduction and codesign in healthcare improvement. *Medical Humanit* 2019; 45: 247–57. http://dx.doi.org/10.1136/medhum-2017-011398.

106. Bate SP, Robert G. Towards more user-centric organisational development: lessons from a case study of experience-based design. *J Appl Behav Sci* 2007; 43: 41–66. https://doi.org/10.1177/0021886306297014.

107. Raynor DK, Ismail H, Blenkinsopp A, et al. Experience-based co-design – adapting the method for a researcher-initiated study in a multi-site setting. *Health Expect* 2020; 23: 562–70. https://doi.org/10.1111/hex.13028.

108. Jones F, Gombert-Waldron K, Honey S, et al. Using co-production to increase activity in acute stroke units: the CREATE mixed-methods study. *Health Serv Deliv Res* 2020; 8(35). https://doi.org/10.3310/hsdr08350.

109. Dixon-Woods M, McNicol S, Martin G. Ten challenges in improving quality in healthcare: lessons from the Health Foundation's programme evaluations and relevant literature. *BMJ Qual Saf* 2012; 21: 876–84. https://doi.org/10.1136/bmjqs-2011-000760.

110. Robert G, MacDonald A. Co-design, organizational creativity and quality improvement in the healthcare sector: 'designerly' or 'design-like?'. In: Sangiorgi D, Prendiville A, editors. *Designing for Service. Contemporary Issues and Novel Spaces*. London: Bloomsbury; 2017: 117–30.

111. Mulgan G, Breckon J, Tarrega M, et al. *Public Value: How Can It be Measured, Managed and Grown?* London: Nesta; 2019. https://media.nesta.org.uk/documents/Public_Value_WEB.pdf (accessed 17 February 2022).

112. Bovaird T, Flemig S, Loeffler E, Osborne SP. How far have we come with co-production – and what's next? *Publ Money Manag* 2019; 39: 229–32. https://doi.org/10.1080/09540962.2019.1592903.

113. Co-production Network for Wales. https://copronet.wales (accessed 17 February 2022).

114. Scottish Co-production Network. www.coproductionscotland.org.uk (accessed 17 February 2022).

115. Q. Special Interest Group. Co-production. https://q.health.org.uk/community/groups/co-production (accessed 17 February 2022).

116. International Coproduction Health Network (ICoHN). http://icohn.org (accessed 17 February 2022).

117. Loeffler E, Bovaird T, editors. *The Palgrave Handbook of Co-Production of Public Services and Outcomes*. London: Palgrave Macmillan; 2021. https://doi.org/10.1007/978-3-030-53705-0.

118. IDEO.org. Design kit. www.designkit.org/methods (accessed 17 February 2022).

Cambridge Elements ≡

Improving Quality and Safety in Healthcare

Editors-in-Chief

Mary Dixon-Woods
THIS Institute (The Healthcare Improvement Studies Institute)

Mary is Director of THIS Institute and is the Health Foundation Professor of Healthcare Improvement Studies in the Department of Public Health and Primary Care at the University of Cambridge. Mary leads a programme of research focused on healthcare improvement, healthcare ethics, and methodological innovation in studying healthcare.

Graham Martin
THIS Institute (The Healthcare Improvement Studies Institute)

Graham is Director of Research at THIS Institute, leading applied research programmes and contributing to the institute's strategy and development. His research interests are in the organisation and delivery of healthcare, and particularly the role of professionals, managers, and patients and the public in efforts at organisational change.

Executive Editor

Katrina Brown
THIS Institute (The Healthcare Improvement Studies Institute)

Katrina is Communications Manager at THIS Institute, providing editorial expertise to maximise the impact of THIS Institute's research findings. She managed the project to produce the series.

Editorial Team

Sonja Marjanovic
RAND Europe

Sonja is Director of RAND Europe's healthcare innovation, industry, and policy research. Her work provides decision-makers with evidence and insights to support innovation and improvement in healthcare systems, and to support the translation of innovation into societal benefits for healthcare services and population health.

Tom Ling
RAND Europe

Tom is Head of Evaluation at RAND Europe and President of the European Evaluation Society, leading evaluations and applied research focused on the key challenges facing health services. His current health portfolio includes evaluations of the innovation landscape, quality improvement, communities of practice, patient flow, and service transformation.

Ellen Perry
THIS Institute (The Healthcare Improvement Studies Institute)
Ellen supported the production of the series during 2020–21.

About the Series

The past decade has seen enormous growth in both activity and research on improvement in healthcare. This series offers a comprehensive and authoritative set of overviews of the different improvement approaches available, exploring the thinking behind them, examining evidence for each approach, and identifying areas of debate.

Cambridge Elements ≡

Improving Quality and Safety in Healthcare

Elements in the Series

Collaboration-Based Approaches
Graham Martin and Mary Dixon-Woods

Co-Producing and Co-Designing
Glenn Robert, Louise Locock, Oli Williams, Jocelyn Cornwell, Sara Donetto, and Joanna Goodrich

The Positive Deviance Approach
Ruth Baxter and Rebecca Lawton

A full series listing is available at: www.cambridge.org/IQ

Printed in the United States
by Baker & Taylor Publisher Services